ENDOMORPH

DIET COOKBOOK FOR SENIOR WOMEN

Boost your Metabolism with a list of food to eat and over 50 Delicious Recipes

Dr. MURAT OZTURK

TABLE OF CONTENTS

Chapter 1

INTRODUCTION

Introduction to endomorph diet

The endomorph diet is designed to cater to the unique metabolic needs of individuals with an endomorph body type. This body type is characterized by a higher percentage of body fat, a wider waist, and a tendency to gain weight easily, particularly in the lower abdomen, hips, and thighs. Understanding and addressing these characteristics can be crucial, especially for senior women who may face additional challenges related to metabolism and hormonal changes.

Senior women with an endomorph body type often find it difficult to lose weight and keep it off due to their naturally slower metabolism and higher fat storage tendency. The endomorph diet focuses on managing these issues by emphasizing a balanced intake of macronutrients that can help boost metabolism, maintain energy levels, and support overall health. Typically, this diet involves a higher proportion of protein and healthy fats while reducing carbohydrate intake, especially refined carbs and sugars. Protein helps in building and maintaining muscle mass, which is essential for boosting metabolism, while healthy fats provide sustained energy and promote satiety, preventing overeating.

For senior women, adopting an endomorph diet can lead to improved energy levels, better blood sugar control, and a lower risk of chronic diseases like diabetes and heart disease. Incorporating regular physical activity, particularly strength training, and moderate cardio, can further enhance the benefits of the diet by increasing muscle mass and promoting fat loss.

Understanding the Endomorph Body Type

Endomorphs typically have a higher percentage of body fat, a wider waist, and a predisposition to easily gain weight. This body type often exhibits a rounded physique with a soft, stocky appearance. Individuals with this body type tend to have a slower metabolism, which means they store fat more readily and find it more challenging to lose weight compared to other body types.

This propensity for fat storage, particularly around the lower abdomen, hips, and thighs, can be attributed to both genetic and hormonal factors. For senior women, these challenges can be compounded by age-related metabolic slowdown and hormonal changes, such as decreased estrogen levels, which further promote fat accumulation and make weight management more difficult.

Endomorphs also often experience higher levels of insulin resistance, which means their bodies do not efficiently use carbohydrates for energy. This inefficiency can lead to increased fat storage when consuming high-carb diets. Therefore, understanding the endomorph body type is essential in developing an effective dietary plan that minimizes carbohydrate intake and emphasizes proteins and healthy fats, which can help manage weight and improve metabolic function.

By understanding the specific needs and characteristics of the endomorph body type, senior women can adopt more personalized and effective strategies for achieving their health and fitness goals. This understanding paves the way for a balanced approach that considers dietary adjustments, exercise routines, and psychological support, ultimately leading to a healthier and more sustainable lifestyle.

Benefits of the Endomorph Diet for Senior Women

One of the primary benefits of the endomorph diet is its emphasis on higher protein intake and healthy fats while reducing carbohydrates, particularly refined carbs, and sugars. This dietary approach helps to stabilize blood sugar levels and reduce insulin resistance, which is often more pronounced in endomorphs. By managing blood sugar levels, senior women can experience improved energy levels and a reduced risk of developing type 2 diabetes.

The diet's focus on whole, unprocessed foods, such as lean proteins, vegetables, and healthy fats, provides essential nutrients that support bodily functions and enhance overall health. These nutrient-dense foods are rich in vitamins, minerals, and antioxidants, which are crucial for maintaining health and preventing age-related diseases. For example, the inclusion of leafy greens, nuts, and fatty fish can help reduce inflammation and promote heart health.

Additionally, the endomorph diet can aid in weight management by promoting satiety and preventing overeating. Healthy fats and proteins take longer to digest, keeping senior women feeling fuller for longer periods. This can help reduce the likelihood of snacking on unhealthy foods and support gradual, sustainable weight loss or maintenance.

Furthermore, by reducing carbohydrate intake, the endomorph diet helps minimize the storage of excess fat, particularly around the midsection, hips, and thighs, which are common trouble spots for endomorphs. This can lead to a more balanced and leaner body composition, improving mobility and reducing the risk of obesity-related conditions.

Chapter 2

UNDERSTANDING ENDOMORPH DIET

The Basics of the Endomorph Diet

The endomorph diet is specifically tailored to address the unique metabolic characteristics of individuals with an endomorph body type, who typically have a higher propensity for fat storage and a slower metabolism. Understanding the basics of this diet is essential for optimizing health and achieving weight management goals, particularly for senior women.

At its core, the endomorph diet focuses on a balanced intake of macronutrients, with an emphasis on higher protein and healthy fat consumption while limiting carbohydrate intake. Protein is a crucial component because it helps build and maintain muscle mass, which is vital for boosting metabolism and burning calories more efficiently. Sources of lean protein such as chicken, turkey, fish, tofu, and legumes are staples in this diet. Healthy fats, derived from foods like avocados, nuts, seeds, and olive oil, provide sustained energy and help promote satiety, reducing the likelihood of overeating.

Carbohydrate intake, especially from refined carbs and sugars, is minimized in the endomorph diet to manage insulin levels and prevent excessive fat storage. Instead, the diet encourages the consumption of complex carbohydrates with a low glycemic index, such as whole grains, vegetables, and fruits, which release glucose more slowly into the bloodstream, providing steady energy without spiking blood sugar levels.

In addition to macronutrient balance, the endomorph diet emphasizes the importance of consuming whole, unprocessed foods. Processed foods often contain added sugars, unhealthy fats, and preservatives that can hinder weight loss and overall health. By focusing on fresh, natural foods, individuals can ensure they are getting essential nutrients, vitamins, and minerals needed for optimal body function. Meal timing and portion control are also significant aspects of the endomorph diet. Eating smaller, more frequent meals throughout the day can help stabilize blood sugar levels and prevent the body from entering a fat-storage mode. This approach helps keep metabolism active and supports sustained energy levels.

Hydration is another critical element of the endomorph diet. Drinking plenty of water throughout the day aids in digestion helps flush out toxins, and can reduce feelings of hunger, contributing to better weight management.

For senior women, incorporating regular physical activity alongside the endomorph diet can enhance its benefits. Strength training and cardiovascular exercises can help build muscle mass, increase metabolic rate, and promote overall health.

Essential Nutrients for Senior Women

The endomorph diet for senior women emphasizes certain essential nutrients that are particularly important for this demographic.

• **Protein** is vital for maintaining muscle mass and strength, which naturally decline with age. Adequate protein intake supports muscle repair and growth, aiding in the maintenance of a healthy metabolism and overall physical function. Lean protein sources such as chicken, fish, beans, and tofu are ideal.

- **Calcium and Vitamin D** are crucial for bone health. Osteoporosis and bone density loss are common concerns for senior women, making these nutrients essential for maintaining strong bones and reducing the risk of fractures. Dairy products, fortified plant-based milk, leafy greens, and supplements are good sources.

- **Healthy fats**, including omega-3 fatty acids, play a significant role in heart health and cognitive function. These fats help reduce inflammation and support brain health, which is particularly important for preventing cognitive decline. Sources include fatty fish like salmon, walnuts, flaxseeds, and olive oil.

•   **Fiber** is essential for digestive health and maintaining stable blood sugar levels. It also aids in weight management by promoting satiety. Senior women should include plenty of high-fiber foods in their diet, such as whole grains, fruits, vegetables, and legumes.

•   **B vitamins**, particularly B6, B12, and folate, are important for energy production, brain health, and the maintenance of red blood cells. These vitamins help prevent anemia and support overall vitality. Foods rich in B vitamins include meat, fish, eggs, dairy products, and leafy greens.

•   **Antioxidants**, such as vitamins C and E, help combat oxidative stress and support immune function. These nutrients can protect against age-related damage and improve skin health. Citrus fruits, berries, nuts, seeds, and colorful vegetables are excellent sources of antioxidants.

• **Magnesium** is involved in over 300 biochemical reactions in the body, including muscle function, bone health, and energy production. It's also important for maintaining normal blood pressure. Foods rich in magnesium include nuts, seeds, whole grains, and green leafy vegetables.

• **Iron** is essential for preventing anemia and maintaining energy levels. Although the need for iron decreases after menopause, it's still important to include iron-rich foods like lean meats, beans, and fortified cereals.

- **Potassium** helps regulate blood pressure and supports heart and muscle function. Senior women should ensure they consume potassium-rich foods such as bananas, sweet potatoes, and spinach.

Characteristics of an endomorph diet

Here are the key characteristics of an endomorph diet:

- **High Protein Intake**: Protein is a cornerstone of the endomorph diet because it helps build and maintain muscle mass, which is crucial for boosting metabolism. Adequate protein intake also promotes satiety, reducing the likelihood of overeating. Lean protein sources such as chicken, turkey, fish, eggs, and plant-based options like beans and tofu are emphasized.

- **Healthy Fats**: Incorporating healthy fats is essential for providing sustained energy and promoting satiety. These fats also support heart health and reduce inflammation. Sources of healthy fats include avocados, nuts, seeds, olive oil, and fatty fish like salmon and mackerel.

- **Low Carbohydrate Intake**: To manage insulin levels and reduce fat storage, the endomorph diet limits carbohydrate intake, especially refined carbs and sugars. Instead, it focuses on complex carbohydrates with a low glycemic index, such as whole grains, vegetables, and fruits.

- **Whole, Unprocessed Foods**: The diet emphasizes the consumption of whole, unprocessed foods to ensure a rich intake of essential nutrients, vitamins, and minerals. Avoiding processed foods helps reduce the intake of added sugars, unhealthy fats, and preservatives that can hinder weight loss and overall health.

• **Balanced Macronutrients**: The endomorph diet seeks to balance macronutrient intake, with a higher proportion of proteins and fats compared to carbohydrates. This balance helps stabilize blood sugar levels, boost metabolism, and maintain energy levels throughout the day.

• **Portion Control and Meal Timing**: To prevent overeating and promote stable blood sugar levels, the diet encourages eating smaller, more frequent meals. This approach keeps metabolism active and prevents the body from entering a fat-storage mode.

• **Hydration**: Drinking plenty of water is a key aspect of the endomorph diet.

Proper hydration aids in digestion, helps flush out toxins and can reduce feelings of hunger, contributing to better weight management.

•	**Regular Physical Activity**: While not strictly a dietary characteristic, incorporating regular physical activity, especially strength training and cardiovascular exercises, enhances the benefits of the endomorph diet.

•	**Customization and Flexibility**: The endomorph diet is adaptable to individual needs and preferences. It can be customized based on specific dietary requirements, health conditions, and lifestyle factors, making it a sustainable and personalized approach to healthy eating.

Chapter 3

ENDOMORPH BODY TYPE EXERCISE FOR SENIORS

Importance of exercise for seniors

Exercise is important for seniors for a variety of reasons, including:

• Maintaining Physical Health: Regular exercise can help seniors maintain physical health by improving muscle strength, flexibility, and balance. This can reduce the risk of falls and injuries, as well as improve cardiovascular health and reduce the risk of chronic diseases such as heart disease and diabetes.

• Improving Mental Health: Exercise can also have a positive impact on mental health, reducing symptoms of depression and anxiety, and improving overall mood and well-being.

27

- Social Interaction: Exercise can provide an opportunity for social interaction and can help seniors stay connected with others, reducing feelings of isolation and loneliness.

- Cognitive Function: Regular exercise has been linked to improved cognitive function, including memory and learning.

- Quality of Life: Regular exercise can improve the overall quality of life for seniors, by promoting independence, increasing energy levels, and improving overall physical and mental health.

Benefits of regular exercise

Regular exercise provides a multitude of benefits for both physical and mental health. Here are some of the key benefits of regular exercise:

- Improved cardiovascular health: Exercise helps to strengthen the heart and circulatory system, reducing the risk of heart disease, stroke, and other cardiovascular conditions.

- Weight management: Exercise helps to burn calories and build muscle mass, aiding in weight management and reducing the risk of obesity and related conditions.

- Increased muscle strength and flexibility: Regular exercise can improve muscle strength, flexibility, and endurance, helping to prevent age-related decline in physical function.

- Improved bone density: Weight-bearing exercise helps to improve bone density, reducing the risk of osteoporosis and related conditions.

- Reduced risk of chronic diseases: Exercise has been shown to reduce the risk of chronic conditions such as type 2 diabetes, high blood pressure, and some types of cancer.

- Improved mental health: Exercise releases endorphins, which can help to improve mood and reduce stress, anxiety, and depression.

- Improved cognitive function: Exercise has been linked to improved cognitive function, including better memory, attention, and problem-solving skills.

- Improved sleep: Exercise can help to regulate sleep patterns, leading to better quality sleep and improved overall health.

Overall, regular exercise is essential for maintaining physical and mental health throughout life, especially as we age.

Challenges faced by seniors with endomorphic body type during exercise

Seniors with endomorphic body type may face several challenges during exercise due to their body type, such as:

•   Difficulty losing weight: Endomorphic body types tend to have a slower metabolism and a tendency to store fat, making it harder to lose weight.

•   Joint pain: Endomorphic body types may be more prone to joint pain and arthritis, which can make exercise more challenging and uncomfortable.

•   Reduced mobility: Endomorphic body types tend to have a larger body size and may have reduced mobility, making certain exercises more difficult or uncomfortable.

• Cardiovascular strain: Carrying excess weight can put additional strain on the cardiovascular system, making certain types of exercise more challenging and potentially dangerous.

• Risk of injury: Seniors with endomorphic body type may have weaker muscles and reduced flexibility, putting them at greater risk of injury during exercise.

Types of exercises suitable for endomorphic body type seniors

Endomorphic body type seniors can benefit from a variety of exercises, including:

• Strength training: Resistance training is particularly beneficial for endomorphic body type seniors as it helps to build muscle mass, which can boost metabolism and aid in weight management. Examples of strength training exercises include bodyweight exercises like squats, lunges, push-ups, and planks, as well as exercises with free weights, resistance bands, or weight machines.

• Cardiovascular exercise: Cardiovascular exercise is important for heart health and weight management. Low-impact exercises such as walking, cycling, swimming, and water aerobics are suitable for endomorphic body type seniors as they reduce the risk of joint pain and injury.

• Flexibility and balance training: Flexibility and balance training are important for maintaining mobility and reducing the risk of falls. Endomorphic body type seniors can benefit from exercises such as yoga, tai chi, or Pilates, which focus on stretching, balance, and core strength.

- Low-impact sports: Sports like golf, pickleball, and bocce ball are low-impact and can provide a fun and social way to stay active.

It's important to start gradually and progress slowly with any exercise program to avoid injury and ensure a sustainable routine. Working with a certified fitness trainer or physical therapist can help endomorphic body type seniors design a safe and effective exercise program tailored to their individual needs and abilities.

Chapter 4

EXERCISE FOR ENDOMORPH SENIORS

Importance of Exercise for Endomorph Seniors

•   Weight management: Endomorph seniors tend to have a slower metabolism and a tendency to store fat, making weight management more challenging. Exercise can help to boost metabolism, burn calories, and build muscle mass, which can aid in weight management and improve overall health.

•   Improved cardiovascular health: Regular exercise helps to strengthen the heart and circulatory system, reducing the risk of heart disease, stroke, and other cardiovascular conditions.

• Improved muscle strength and flexibility: Exercise helps to improve muscle strength, flexibility, and endurance, reducing the risk of age-related decline in physical function.

• Improved bone density: Weight-bearing exercise helps to improve bone density, reducing the risk of osteoporosis and related conditions.

• Reduced risk of chronic diseases: Exercise has been shown to reduce the risk of chronic conditions such as type 2 diabetes, high blood pressure, and some types of cancer.

• Improved mental health: Exercise releases endorphins, which can help to improve mood and reduce stress, anxiety, and depression.

•   Improved cognitive function: Exercise has been linked to improved cognitive function, including better memory, attention, and problem-solving skills.

•   Improved sleep: Exercise can help to regulate sleep patterns, leading to better quality sleep and improved overall health.

Best exercises for endomorph seniors

Endomorph seniors can benefit from a variety of exercises, including:

•   Low-impact cardio exercises: Endomorph seniors can benefit from low-impact cardio exercises that are easy on the joints such as walking, swimming, cycling, water aerobics, or using an elliptical machine. These exercises can help to burn calories, boost metabolism, and improve cardiovascular health.

• Strength training exercises: Strength training exercises can help endomorph seniors build muscle mass, which can boost metabolism and aid in weight management. Bodyweight exercises like squats, lunges, push-ups, and planks, as well as exercises with free weights, resistance bands, or weight machines, can be suitable for endomorph seniors.

• Flexibility and balance exercises: Endomorph seniors can benefit from exercises that improve flexibility and balance such as yoga, Pilates, and Tai Chi. These exercises can help to reduce the risk of falls and improve overall mobility.

• Low-impact sports: Endomorph seniors can also participate in low-impact sports such as golf, pickleball, or bocce ball, which provide a fun and social way to stay active.

Endomorph seniors need to start gradually and progress slowly with any exercise program to avoid injury and ensure a sustainable routine.

Resistance training for endomorph seniors

Resistance training, also known as strength training, is an excellent exercise option for endomorph seniors. Resistance training involves using resistance to build muscle strength, improve bone density, and boost metabolism.

Here are some key tips for resistance training for endomorph seniors:

•   Start gradually: It's essential to start with light weights or resistance bands and gradually increase the intensity, weight, or resistance over time.

- **Focus on form:** Proper form is crucial to avoid injury and get the most benefit from resistance training. Seniors should work with a certified fitness trainer to ensure proper form and technique.

- **Train all major muscle groups:** Resistance training should target all major muscle groups, including the arms, chest, back, legs, and core.

- **Use a variety of exercises:** Using a variety of exercises can help to prevent boredom and target different muscle groups. Some examples of resistance exercises include bicep curls, tricep extensions, chest presses, leg presses, squats, and lunges.

- **Allow for adequate rest and recovery:** Rest is essential for muscle recovery and growth. Seniors should avoid overtraining and allow for adequate rest between resistance training sessions.

•   Incorporate resistance training into a well-rounded exercise program: Resistance training should be part of a well-rounded exercise program that includes cardio, flexibility, and balance exercises.

In conclusion, resistance training can be a safe and effective exercise option for endomorph seniors when done correctly.

Cardiovascular exercise for endomorph seniors

Cardiovascular exercise, also known as cardio, is an essential component of any exercise program, especially for endomorph seniors. Cardio exercises increase the heart rate, improve lung capacity, burn calories, and strengthen the cardiovascular system.

Here are some key tips for cardiovascular exercise for endomorph seniors:

• Start gradually: It's essential to start with low-intensity cardio exercises and gradually increase the intensity, duration, and frequency over time. Walking, swimming, and cycling are great low-intensity cardio options for endomorph seniors.

• Choose low-impact exercises: Endomorph seniors should choose low-impact exercises that are easy on the joints to avoid injury. Water aerobics, using an elliptical machine, or using a stationary bike are good options.

• Monitor heart rate: Endomorph seniors should monitor their heart rate during cardio exercises to ensure they're working at a safe and effective level. A target heart rate range can be calculated based on age and fitness level.

•	Mix it up: Variety is essential to avoid boredom and challenge the cardiovascular system in different ways. Endomorph seniors should mix up their cardio exercises with different types, such as walking one day and swimming the next.

•	Incorporate interval training: Interval training involves alternating between periods of high-intensity exercise and rest or low-intensity exercise. This type of training can help to boost metabolism, burn calories, and improve cardiovascular fitness. For example, an endomorph senior could walk at a brisk pace for one minute, then slow down to a leisurely pace for two minutes, and repeat.

- Aim for at least 150 minutes of moderate-intensity cardio per week: The American Heart Association recommends that adults aim for at least 150 minutes of moderate-intensity cardio per week. This can be divided into several sessions throughout the week.

Cardiovascular exercise is an important component of any exercise program for endomorph seniors. It's important to choose low-impact exercises, monitor heart rate, and gradually increase intensity and duration over time. Working with a certified fitness trainer can help endomorph seniors design a safe and effective cardio program tailored to their individual needs and abilities

Chapter 5

ENDOMORPH BODY TYPE FOOD LIST

Comprehensive food list to eat

Proteins:

1. **Fish:**

    - Salmon

    - Mackerel

    - Sardines

    - Trout

2. **Lean Meats:**

    - Chicken breast

    - Turkey

    - Lean cuts of beef or pork

3. **Dairy:**

- Greek yogurt (low-fat or fat-free)

- Cottage cheese

- Eggs

4. **Plant-Based Proteins:**

- Lentils

- Chickpeas

- Quinoa

- Tofu

- Edamame

5. **Nuts and Seeds:**

- Almonds

- Walnuts

- Chia seeds

- Flaxseeds

Vegetables:

1. **Leafy Greens:**

   - Spinach

   - Kale

   - Swiss chard

   - Collard greens

2. **Colorful Vegetables:**

   - Broccoli

   - Bell peppers

   - Carrots

   - Tomatoes

3. **Cruciferous Vegetables:**

   - Cauliflower

   - Brussels sprouts

- Cabbage

4. **Root Vegetables:**

   - Sweet potatoes

   - Carrots

   - Beets

5. **Legumes:**

   - Beans (black beans, kidney beans, chickpeas)

   - Lentils

Fruits:

1. **Berries:**

   - Blueberries

   - Strawberries

   - Raspberries

2. **Citrus Fruits:**

    - Oranges

    - Grapefruits

    - Lemons

3. **Bananas**

4. **Apples**

5. **Avocado**

Whole Grains:

1. Quinoa

2. Brown rice

3. Oats

4. Barley

5. Whole grain bread and pasta

Healthy Fats:

1. Olive oil

2. Avocado

3. Nuts and seeds

4. Fatty fish (salmon, mackerel)

5. Flaxseed oil

Dairy or Dairy Alternatives:

1. Low-fat or fat-free milk

2. Low-fat or fat-free yogurt

3. Cheese in moderation

Fluids:

1. Water

2. Herbal teas

3. Low-sodium vegetable juice

Snacks:

1. Fresh fruit slices

2. Vegetable sticks with hummus

3. Greek yogurt with berries

4. Nuts and seeds mix

Herbs and Spices:

1. Turmeric

2. Cinnamon

3. Ginger

4. Garlic

5. Oregano

Supplements (as advised by a healthcare professional):

1. Calcium and Vitamin D for bone health

2. Omega-3 fatty acids

3. Multivitamins

Comprehensive list of foods to avoid

Processed and Sugary Foods:

1. Sodas and sugary drinks

2. Candy and sweets

3. Commercially baked goods (cakes, pastries, cookies)

4. Processed cereals with added sugars

Refined Carbohydrates:

1. White bread

2. White rice

3. White pasta

4. Refined breakfast cereals

Fried and Fast Foods:

1. French fries

2. Fried chicken

3. Fast food burgers and fries

4. Processed and fried snacks (potato chips, nachos)

High-Fat Meats:

1. Fatty cuts of red meat

2. Processed meats (sausages, hot dogs, bacon)

3. Fried and breaded meats

Full-Fat Dairy:

1. Full-fat milk

2. Full-fat cheese

3. Cream and butter in excess

High-Sugar and High-Fat Sauces:

1. Sweetened ketchup

2. Barbecue sauce with added sugars

3. Creamy and high-fat salad dressings

Highly Processed Snacks:

1. Packaged snacks with high sugar and fat content

2. Microwave popcorn with added butter

3. Processed cheese snacks

Alcohol:

1. Excessive alcohol consumption

2. Sweetened and high-calorie cocktails

Salty and High-Sodium Foods:

1. Processed and canned soups with high-sodium

2. Canned and processed meats

3. Excessively salty snacks (pretzels, salted nuts)

Sweetened and Flavored Beverages:

1. Sweetened fruit juices

2. Energy drinks

3. Flavored coffee drinks with added sugars

Artificial Sweeteners and Diet Products:

1. Diet sodas with artificial sweeteners

2. Sugar-free candies with artificial sweeteners

Highly Processed and Convenience Foods:

1. Frozen meals with high sodium and additives

2. Instant noodles and packaged convenience foods

3. Highly processed and pre-packaged meals

Considerations for Seniors:

1. Limit caffeine intake, especially in the evening.

2. Be cautious with spicy foods if they cause digestive discomfort.

3. Monitor portion sizes to avoid overeating.

Chapter 6

ENDOMORPH BREAKFAST RECIPES

Protein-Packed Scrambled Eggs

Ingredients:
- 2 eggs
- 1/4 cup diced vegetables (bell peppers, onions, spinach)
- 1 tablespoon olive oil
- Salt and pepper to taste

Instructions:
1. Heat olive oil in a non-stick skillet over medium heat.
2. Add diced vegetables and sauté until softened.
3. Beat eggs in a bowl and pour into the skillet with the vegetables.
4. Cook, stirring occasionally, until eggs are scrambled and cooked through.
5. Season with salt and pepper.

6. Serve hot.

Nutritional Information (per serving):

- Calories: 220

- Protein: 12g

- Fat: 16g

- Carbohydrates: 6g

Greek Yogurt Parfait

Ingredients:

- 1/2 cup Greek yogurt

- 1/4 cup mixed berries (strawberries, blueberries, raspberries)

- 2 tablespoons granola

- 1 teaspoon honey (optional)

Instructions:

1. In a serving glass or bowl, layer Greek yogurt, mixed berries, and granola.

2. Drizzle with honey if desired.

3. Repeat layers if necessary.

4. Serve immediately.

Nutritional Information (per serving):

- Calories: 200
- Protein: 15g
- Fat: 6g
- Carbohydrates: 25g

Avocado Toast with Poached Eggs

Ingredients:

- 1 slice whole grain bread
- 1/2 avocado, mashed
- 1 poached egg
- Salt and pepper to taste

Instructions:

1. Toast the whole-grain bread until golden brown.
2. Spread mashed avocado evenly on the toast.
3. Top with a poached egg.
4. Season with salt and pepper.
5. Serve warm.

Nutritional Information (per serving):

- Calories: 250
- Protein: 11g
- Fat: 15g
- Carbohydrates: 20g

Vegetable Omelette

Ingredients:

- 2 eggs
- 1/4 cup diced vegetables (bell peppers, onions, tomatoes, mushrooms)
- 1 tablespoon olive oil
- Salt and pepper to taste

Instructions:

1. Heat olive oil in a non-stick skillet over medium heat.
2. Add diced vegetables and sauté until tender.

3. Beat eggs in a bowl and pour over the vegetables.

4. Cook until the edges start to set, then gently lift the edges and tilt the pan to let the uncooked egg flow underneath.

5. Once the omelette is mostly set, fold it in half and cook for another minute.

6. Season with salt and pepper.

7. Serve hot.

Nutritional Information (per serving):

- Calories: 220
- Protein: 12g
- Fat: 16g
- Carbohydrates: 6g

Banana Nut Oatmeal

Ingredients:

- 1/2 cup rolled oats
- 1 cup water or milk

- 1/2 banana, sliced
- 1 tablespoon chopped nuts (almonds, walnuts, pecans)
- 1 teaspoon honey (optional)

Instructions:

1. In a saucepan, bring water or milk to a boil.
2. Stir in rolled oats and reduce heat to low.
3. Cook, stirring occasionally, until oats are tender and liquid is absorbed.
4. Transfer oatmeal to a bowl and top with sliced banana and chopped nuts.
5. Drizzle with honey if desired.
6. Serve warm.

Nutritional Information (per serving):

- Calories: 300
- Protein: 10g
- Fat: 8g

- Carbohydrates: 50g

Spinach and Feta Frittata

Ingredients:

- 4 eggs
- 1 cup fresh spinach leaves
- 1/4 cup crumbled feta cheese
- 1/4 cup diced tomatoes
- Salt and pepper to taste

Instructions:

1. Preheat oven to 350°F (175°C).
2. In a bowl, beat eggs and season with salt and pepper.
3. Stir in spinach, feta cheese, and diced tomatoes.
4. Pour the mixture into a greased baking dish.
5. Bake for 20-25 minutes or until set and golden brown on top.
6. Slice into wedges and serve warm.

Nutritional Information (per serving):

- Calories: 220
- Protein: 16g
- Fat: 15g
- Carbohydrates: 5g

Protein Smoothie Bowl

Ingredients:

- 1/2 cup Greek yogurt
- 1/2 frozen banana
- 1/2 cup mixed berries (strawberries, blueberries, raspberries)
- 1 scoop protein powder
- 1/4 cup almond milk
- Toppings: sliced almonds, chia seeds, shredded coconut

Instructions:

1. In a blender, combine Greek yogurt, frozen banana, mixed berries, protein powder, and almond milk.

2. Blend until smooth and creamy.

3. Pour into a bowl and top with sliced almonds, chia seeds, and shredded coconut.

4. Serve immediately with a spoon.

Nutritional Information (per serving):

- Calories: 300

- Protein: 25g

- Fat: 8g

- Carbohydrates: 30g

Whole Grain Pancakes with Berries

Ingredients:

- 1/2 cup whole wheat flour

- 1/2 teaspoon baking powder

- 1/4 teaspoon cinnamon

- 1/2 cup milk (or almond milk)

- 1 egg

- 1 tablespoon honey (optional)

- Mixed berries for topping

Instructions:

1. In a bowl, whisk together whole wheat flour, baking powder, and cinnamon.
2. In another bowl, beat together milk, egg, and honey (if using).
3. Pour wet ingredients into dry ingredients and stir until just combined.
4. Heat a non-stick skillet over medium heat and lightly grease with cooking spray.
5. Pour batter onto the skillet to form pancakes.
6. Cook until bubbles form on the surface, then flip and cook until golden brown on the other side.
7. Serve pancakes topped with mixed berries.

Nutritional Information (per serving):

- Calories: 250
- Protein: 10g
- Fat: 5g
- Carbohydrates: 40g

Vegetable Breakfast Burrito

Ingredients:

- 1 whole grain tortilla
- 2 eggs, scrambled
- 1/4 cup black beans, drained and rinsed
- 2 tablespoons salsa
- 1/4 avocado, sliced
- Handful of spinach leaves
- Salt and pepper to taste

Instructions:

1. Heat the tortilla in a dry skillet until warmed through.

2. Fill the tortilla with scrambled eggs, black beans, salsa, avocado slices, and spinach leaves.

3. Season with salt and pepper.

4. Roll up the tortilla to form a burrito.

5. Serve warm.

Nutritional Information (per serving):

- Calories: 320

- Protein: 18g

- Fat: 15g

- Carbohydrates: 30g

Quinoa Breakfast Bowl

Ingredients:

- 1/2 cup cooked quinoa

- 1/4 cup Greek yogurt

- 1/4 cup mixed berries (strawberries, blueberries, raspberries)

- 1 tablespoon chopped nuts (almonds, walnuts, pecans)

- 1 teaspoon honey (optional)

Instructions:

1. In a bowl, layer cooked quinoa, Greek yogurt, mixed berries, and chopped nuts.
2. Drizzle with honey if desired.
3. Serve warm or chilled.

Nutritional Information (per serving):

- Calories: 280
- Protein: 15g
- Fat: 8g
- Carbohydrates: 40g

Sweet Potato Hash

Ingredients:

- 1 small sweet potato, diced
- 1/4 cup diced bell peppers
- 1/4 cup diced onions
- 2 slices turkey bacon, chopped
- 1 tablespoon olive oil

- Salt and pepper to taste

Instructions:

1. Heat olive oil in a skillet over medium heat.
2. Add diced sweet potato and cook until softened and slightly browned.
3. Add diced bell peppers, onions, and chopped turkey bacon to the skillet.
4. Cook until vegetables are tender and bacon is crispy.
5. Season with salt and pepper.
6. Serve hot.

Nutritional Information (per serving):

- Calories: 280
- Protein: 8g
- Fat: 15g
- Carbohydrates: 30g

Chapter 7

ENDOMORPH LUNCH RECIPES

Grilled Chicken Salad

Ingredients:

- 4 oz grilled chicken breast
- Mixed salad greens
- 1/4 cup cherry tomatoes, halved
- 1/4 cucumber, sliced
- 1/4 avocado, sliced
- Balsamic vinaigrette dressing

Instructions:

1. Grill chicken breast until cooked through.
2. Arrange mixed salad greens on a plate and top with cherry tomatoes, cucumber slices, and avocado.
3. Slice grilled chicken and place on top of the salad.

4. Drizzle with balsamic vinaigrette dressing.

5. Serve immediately.

Nutritional Information (per serving):

- Calories: 300
- Protein: 25g
- Fat: 15g
- Carbohydrates: 15g

Turkey and Veggie Wrap

Ingredients:

- 1 whole-grain tortilla
- 2 slices turkey breast
- 1/4 cup mixed salad greens
- 1/4 cup shredded carrots
- 1/4 cup sliced bell peppers
- 1 tablespoon hummus

Instructions:

1. Lay the whole-grain tortilla flat on a clean surface.

2. Spread hummus evenly over the tortilla.

3. Layer turkey breast, mixed salad greens, shredded carrots, and sliced bell peppers on top of the hummus.

4. Roll up the tortilla tightly.

5. Cut the wrap in half diagonally.

6. Serve immediately.

Nutritional Information (per serving):

- Calories: 250

- Protein: 20g

- Fat: 10g

- Carbohydrates: 25g

Salmon Quinoa Bowl

Ingredients:

- 4 oz baked salmon fillet

- 1/2 cup cooked quinoa

- 1/4 cup steamed broccoli florets

- 1/4 cup sliced bell peppers

- 1/4 cup shredded carrots
- 1 tablespoon olive oil
- Lemon wedge for garnish

Instructions:

1. Preheat oven to 375°F (190°C).
2. Place the salmon fillet on a baking sheet lined with parchment paper.
3. Drizzle olive oil over the salmon and season with salt and pepper.
4. Bake for 15-20 minutes or until salmon is cooked through.
5. In a bowl, layer cooked quinoa, steamed broccoli florets, sliced bell peppers, and shredded carrots.
6. Place baked salmon on top of the quinoa bowl.
7. Garnish with a lemon wedge.
8. Serve warm.

Nutritional Information (per serving):

- Calories: 350

- Protein: 25g

- Fat: 15g

- Carbohydrates: 30g

Tuna Salad Stuffed Avocado

Ingredients:

- 1 ripe avocado

- 1/2 cup canned tuna, drained

- 1 tablespoon Greek yogurt

- 1 tablespoon diced red onion

- 1 tablespoon diced celery

- Salt and pepper to taste

Instructions:

1. Cut the avocado in half and remove the pit.

2. In a bowl, mix canned tuna, Greek yogurt, diced red onion, and diced celery.

3. Season with salt and pepper.

4. Spoon the tuna salad mixture into the avocado halves.

5. Serve immediately.

Nutritional Information (per serving):

- Calories: 300

- Protein: 20g

- Fat: 20g

- Carbohydrates: 10g

Vegetable and Lentil Soup

Ingredients:

- 1/2 cup cooked lentils

- 1 cup mixed vegetables (carrots, celery, onions, zucchini)

- 2 cups vegetable broth

- 1 tablespoon olive oil

- Salt and pepper to taste

Instructions:

1. Heat olive oil in a pot over medium heat.

2. Add mixed vegetables and sauté until softened.

3. Add cooked lentils and vegetable broth to the pot.

4. Bring to a boil, then reduce heat and simmer for 15-20 minutes.

5. Season with salt and pepper.

6. Serve hot.

Nutritional Information (per serving):

- Calories: 250
- Protein: 15g
- Fat: 5g
- Carbohydrates: 40g

Eggplant Parmesan

Ingredients:

- 1 small eggplant, sliced
- 1/4 cup whole wheat bread crumbs
- 1/4 cup grated Parmesan cheese
- 1 cup marinara sauce

- 1/4 cup shredded mozzarella cheese
- Fresh basil leaves for garnish

Instructions:

1. Preheat oven to 375°F (190°C).
2. Dip eggplant slices in whole wheat bread crumbs and grated Parmesan cheese.
3. Place eggplant slices on a baking sheet lined with parchment paper.
4. Bake for 20-25 minutes or until eggplant is tender and golden brown.
5. In a baking dish, spread marinara sauce evenly on the bottom.
6. Place baked eggplant slices on top of the marinara sauce.
7. Sprinkle shredded mozzarella cheese over the eggplant.
8. Bake for an additional 10 minutes or until cheese is melted and bubbly.

9. Garnish with fresh basil leaves.

10. Serve hot.

Nutritional Information (per serving):

- Calories: 300

- Protein: 15g

- Fat: 10g

- Carbohydrates: 35g

Chicken and Vegetable Stir-Fry

Ingredients:

- 4 oz cooked chicken breast, sliced

- 1 cup mixed vegetables (bell peppers, broccoli, carrots)

- 1 tablespoon olive oil

- 2 tablespoons low-sodium soy sauce

- 1 tablespoon honey

- 1 clove garlic, minced

- 1/2 teaspoon grated ginger

- Cooked brown rice for serving

Instructions:

1. Heat olive oil in a skillet over medium-high heat.
2. Add minced garlic and grated ginger to the skillet and sauté until fragrant.
3. Add mixed vegetables and cooked chicken breast slices to the skillet.
4. Stir-fry for 3-4 minutes or until vegetables are tender-crisp.
5. In a small bowl, whisk together low-sodium soy sauce and honey.
6. Pour the soy sauce mixture over the chicken and vegetables.
7. Stir well to coat evenly.
8. Serve stir-fry over cooked brown rice.

Nutritional Information (per serving):

- Calories: 350
- Protein: 25g
- Fat: 10g
- Carbohydrates: 40g

Quinoa Salad with Chickpeas

Ingredients:

- 1/2 cup cooked quinoa
- 1/2 cup canned chickpeas, drained and rinsed
- 1/4 cup diced cucumber
- 1/4 cup halved cherry tomatoes
- 1/4 cup diced red onion
- 2 tablespoons chopped fresh parsley
- 1 tablespoon olive oil
- 1 tablespoon lemon juice
- Salt and pepper to taste

Instructions:

1. In a bowl, combine cooked quinoa, canned chickpeas, diced cucumber, halved cherry tomatoes, diced red onion, and chopped fresh parsley.
2. Drizzle olive oil and lemon juice over the salad.

3. Season with salt and pepper.

4. Toss gently to combine.

5. Serve chilled or at room temperature.

Nutritional Information (per serving):

- Calories: 300

- Protein: 12g

- Fat: 10g

- Carbohydrates: 40g

Vegetarian Chili

Ingredients:

- 1 can (15 oz) black beans, drained and rinsed

- 1 can (15 oz) kidney beans, drained and rinsed

- 1 can (15 oz) diced tomatoes

- 1 cup vegetable broth

- 1/2 cup diced bell peppers

- 1/2 cup diced onions

- 1/4 cup corn kernels

- 2 cloves garlic, minced
- 1 tablespoon olive oil
- 1 tablespoon chili powder
- 1 teaspoon cumin
- Salt and pepper to taste

Instructions:

1. Heat olive oil in a pot over medium heat.
2. Add minced garlic, diced onions, and diced bell peppers to the pot.
3. Sauté until vegetables are softened.
4. Add black beans, kidney beans, diced tomatoes, vegetable broth, corn kernels, chili powder, cumin, salt, and pepper to the pot.
5. Bring to a boil, then reduce heat and simmer for 20-25 minutes.
6. Serve hot.

Nutritional Information (per serving):

- Calories: 300

- Protein: 15g
- Fat: 5g
- Carbohydrates: 50g

Mediterranean Quinoa Salad

Ingredients:

- 1/2 cup cooked quinoa
- 1/4 cup chopped cucumber
- 1/4 cup halved cherry tomatoes
- 1/4 cup chopped bell peppers
- 1/4 cup diced red onion
- 2 tablespoons crumbled feta cheese
- 2 tablespoons chopped fresh parsley
- 1 tablespoon olive oil
- 1 tablespoon lemon juice
- Salt and pepper to taste

Instructions:

1. In a bowl, combine cooked quinoa, chopped cucumber, halved cherry tomatoes, chopped bell peppers,

diced red onion, crumbled feta cheese, and chopped fresh parsley.

2. Drizzle olive oil and lemon juice over the salad.
3. Season with salt and pepper.
4. Toss gently to combine.
5. Serve chilled or at room temperature.

Nutritional Information (per serving):

- Calories: 250
- Protein: 8g
- Fat: 10g
- Carbohydrates: 35g

Lentil and Vegetable Soup

Ingredients:

- 1/2 cup cooked lentils
- 2 cups mixed vegetables (carrots, celery, onions, potatoes)
- 4 cups vegetable broth
- 1 tablespoon olive oil

- 2 cloves garlic, minced
- 1/2 teaspoon dried thyme
- Salt and pepper to taste

Instructions:

1. Heat olive oil in a pot over medium heat.
2. Add minced garlic to the pot and sauté until fragrant.
3. Add mixed vegetables and dried thyme to the pot.
4. Cook for 5 minutes, stirring occasionally.
5. Add cooked lentils and vegetable broth to the pot.
6. Bring to a boil, then reduce heat and simmer for 20-25 minutes.
7. Season with salt and pepper.
8. Serve hot.

Nutritional Information (per serving):

- Calories: 250

- Protein: 10g

- Fat: 5g

- Carbohydrates: 40g

Mushroom and Spinach Quesadilla

Ingredients:

- 2 whole grain tortillas

- 1 cup sliced mushrooms

- 1 cup fresh spinach leaves

- 1/2 cup shredded mozzarella cheese

- 1/4 cup sliced onions

- 1/4 cup sliced bell peppers

- 1 tablespoon olive oil

- Salsa and Greek yogurt for dipping

Instructions:

1. Heat olive oil in a skillet over medium heat.

2. Add sliced mushrooms, onions, and bell peppers to the skillet.

3. Sauté until vegetables are softened.

4. Remove vegetables from the skillet and set aside.

5. Place one whole-grain tortilla in the skillet.

6. Layer shredded mozzarella cheese, sautéed vegetables, and fresh spinach leaves on top of the tortilla.

7. Place the second tortilla on top.

8. Cook until the bottom tortilla is golden brown and crispy.

9. Carefully flip the quesadilla and cook until the other side is golden brown and crispy.

10. Remove from the skillet and cut into wedges.

11. Serve hot with salsa and Greek yogurt for dipping.

Nutritional Information (per serving):

- Calories: 350
- Protein: 15g

- Fat: 15g
- Carbohydrates: 40g

Chapter 8

ENDOMORPH DINNER RECIPES

Baked Salmon with Roasted Vegetables

Ingredients:

- 4 oz salmon fillet
- 1 cup mixed vegetables (bell peppers, zucchini, carrots)
- 1 tablespoon olive oil
- Salt and pepper to taste
- Lemon wedges for garnish

Instructions:

1. Preheat oven to 375°F (190°C).
2. Place the salmon fillet on a baking sheet lined with parchment paper.
3. Toss mixed vegetables with olive oil, salt, and pepper.
4. Arrange vegetables around the salmon on the baking sheet.

5. Bake for 15-20 minutes or until salmon is cooked through and vegetables are tender.

6. Serve hot with lemon wedges.

Nutritional Information (per serving):

- Calories: 300
- Protein: 25g
- Fat: 15g
- Carbohydrates: 15g

Turkey Meatballs with Whole Wheat Pasta

Ingredients:

- 4 oz ground turkey
- 1/4 cup whole wheat bread crumbs
- 1/4 cup grated Parmesan cheese
- 1 egg
- 1 clove garlic, minced
- 1/4 cup chopped fresh parsley
- 1 cup cooked whole wheat pasta
- 1 cup marinara sauce

Instructions:

1. Preheat oven to 375°F (190°C).
2. In a bowl, mix ground turkey, whole wheat bread crumbs, grated Parmesan cheese, egg, minced garlic, and chopped fresh parsley.
3. Shape the mixture into meatballs and place on a baking sheet lined with parchment paper.
4. Bake for 20-25 minutes or until meatballs are cooked through.
5. Heat marinara sauce in a saucepan over medium heat.
6. Add cooked meatballs to the sauce and simmer for 5 minutes.
7. Serve meatballs and sauce over cooked whole wheat pasta.

Nutritional Information (per serving):

- Calories: 350
- Protein: 25g

- Fat: 15g

- Carbohydrates: 30g

Chicken Stir-Fry with Brown Rice

Ingredients:

- 4 oz cooked chicken breast, sliced
- 1 cup mixed vegetables (bell peppers, broccoli, carrots)
- 1 tablespoon olive oil
- 2 tablespoons low-sodium soy sauce
- 1 tablespoon honey
- 1 clove garlic, minced
- 1/2 teaspoon grated ginger
- 1 cup cooked brown rice

Instructions:

1. Heat olive oil in a skillet over medium-high heat.
2. Add minced garlic and grated ginger to the skillet and sauté until fragrant.

3. Add mixed vegetables and cooked chicken breast slices to the skillet.
4. Stir-fry for 3-4 minutes or until vegetables are tender-crisp.
5. In a small bowl, whisk together low-sodium soy sauce and honey.
6. Pour the soy sauce mixture over the chicken and vegetables.
7. Stir well to coat evenly.
8. Serve stir-fry over cooked brown rice.

Nutritional Information (per serving):

- Calories: 400
- Protein: 25g
- Fat: 15g
- Carbohydrates: 40g

Quinoa Stuffed Bell Peppers

Ingredients:

- 2 bell peppers, halved and seeds removed

- 1/2 cup cooked quinoa
- 1/4 cup black beans, drained and rinsed
- 1/4 cup corn kernels
- 1/4 cup diced tomatoes
- 1/4 cup shredded cheese
- 1 tablespoon chopped fresh cilantro
- Salt and pepper to taste

Instructions:

1. Preheat oven to 375°F (190°C).
2. In a bowl, mix cooked quinoa, black beans, corn kernels, diced tomatoes, shredded cheese, chopped fresh cilantro, salt, and pepper.
3. Stuff each bell pepper half with the quinoa mixture.
4. Place stuffed bell peppers on a baking sheet lined with parchment paper.

5. Bake for 25-30 minutes or until peppers are tender.

6. Serve hot.

Nutritional Information (per serving):

- Calories: 300

- Protein: 15g

- Fat: 10g

- Carbohydrates: 40g

Baked Chicken with Sweet Potato Mash

Ingredients:

- 4 oz chicken breast

- 1 small sweet potato, peeled and diced

- 1 tablespoon olive oil

- Salt and pepper to taste

- Fresh parsley for garnish

Instructions:

1. Preheat oven to 375°F (190°C).

2. Place chicken breast on a baking sheet lined with parchment paper.

3. Drizzle olive oil over the chicken and season with salt and pepper.

4. Bake for 20-25 minutes or until chicken is cooked through.

5. While the chicken is baking, steam or boil diced sweet potato until tender.

6. Mash the cooked sweet potato with a fork until smooth.

7. Serve baked chicken with sweet potato mash.

8. Garnish with fresh parsley.

Nutritional Information (per serving):

- Calories: 300
- Protein: 25g
- Fat: 10g
- Carbohydrates: 25g

Shrimp and Vegetable Stir-Fry

Ingredients:

- 4 oz shrimp, peeled and deveined
- 1 cup mixed vegetables (bell peppers, snap peas, carrots)
- 1 tablespoon olive oil
- 2 tablespoons low-sodium soy sauce
- 1 tablespoon honey
- 1 clove garlic, minced
- 1/2 teaspoon grated ginger
- Cooked brown rice for serving

Instructions:

1. Heat olive oil in a skillet over medium-high heat.
2. Add minced garlic and grated ginger to the skillet and sauté until fragrant.
3. Add mixed vegetables and shrimp to the skillet.

4. Stir-fry for 3-4 minutes or until shrimp are pink and vegetables are tender-crisp.

5. In a small bowl, whisk together low-sodium soy sauce and honey.

6. Pour the soy sauce mixture over the shrimp and vegetables.

7. Stir well to coat evenly.

8. Serve stir-fry over cooked brown rice.

Nutritional Information (per serving):

- Calories: 350

- Protein: 20g

- Fat: 10g

- Carbohydrates: 45g

Mediterranean Chicken Skewers with Greek Salad

Ingredients:

- 4 oz chicken breast, cut into chunks

- 1/4 cup cherry tomatoes

- 1/4 cup cucumber, sliced

- 1/4 cup red onion, sliced
- 2 tablespoons feta cheese, crumbled
- 1 tablespoon olive oil
- 1 tablespoon lemon juice
- 1/2 teaspoon dried oregano
- Salt and pepper to taste

Instructions:

1. Preheat the grill or grill pan over medium-high heat.
2. Thread chicken breast chunks onto skewers.
3. In a bowl, whisk together olive oil, lemon juice, dried oregano, salt, and pepper.
4. Brush the chicken skewers with the olive oil mixture.
5. Grill chicken skewers for 8-10 minutes, turning occasionally, until cooked through.

6. In a separate bowl, combine cherry tomatoes, cucumber, red onion, and crumbled feta cheese to make the Greek salad.

7. Drizzle with olive oil and lemon juice.

8. Season with salt and pepper.

9. Serve grilled chicken skewers with Greek salad.

Nutritional Information (per serving):

- Calories: 350
- Protein: 25g
- Fat: 15g
- Carbohydrates: 20g

Vegetable Stir-Fried Rice

Ingredients:

- 1 cup cooked brown rice
- 1 cup mixed vegetables (bell peppers, broccoli, carrots)
- 2 eggs, lightly beaten

- 2 tablespoons low-sodium soy sauce

- 1 tablespoon olive oil

- 1 clove garlic, minced

- Salt and pepper to taste

- Green onions for garnish

Instructions:

1. Heat olive oil in a skillet over medium heat.

2. Add minced garlic to the skillet and sauté until fragrant.

3. Add mixed vegetables to the skillet and stir-fry until tender-crisp.

4. Push the vegetables to one side of the skillet and pour the beaten eggs into the other side.

5. Scramble the eggs until cooked through, then mix with the vegetables.

6. Add cooked brown rice and low-sodium soy sauce to the skillet.

7. Stir well to combine.

8. Season with salt and pepper.

9. Garnish with chopped green onions.

10. Serve hot.

Nutritional Information (per serving):

- Calories: 300

- Protein: 12g

- Fat: 10g

- Carbohydrates: 40g

Baked Cod with Lemon Herb Sauce

Ingredients:

- 4 oz cod fillet

- 1 tablespoon olive oil

- 1 tablespoon lemon juice

- 1 teaspoon dried herbs (such as thyme, rosemary, or dill)

- Salt and pepper to taste

- Lemon wedges for garnish

Instructions:

1. Preheat oven to 375°F (190°C).
2. Place the cod fillet on a baking sheet lined with parchment paper.
3. Drizzle olive oil and lemon juice over the cod.
4. Sprinkle dried herbs, salt, and pepper over the cod.
5. Bake for 15-20 minutes or until cod is cooked through and flakes easily with a fork.
6. Serve hot with lemon wedges.

Nutritional Information (per serving):

- Calories: 250
- Protein: 25g
- Fat: 10g
- Carbohydrates: 10g

Chapter 9

ENDOMORPH SNACKS RECIPES

Greek Yogurt with Berries

Ingredients:

- 1/2 cup Greek yogurt
- 1/4 cup mixed berries (strawberries, blueberries, raspberries)
- 1 tablespoon honey (optional)

Instructions:

1. Spoon Greek yogurt into a bowl.
2. Top with mixed berries.
3. Drizzle with honey if desired.
4. Serve chilled.

Nutritional Information (per serving):

- Calories: 100
- Protein: 10g
- Fat: 0g
- Carbohydrates: 15g

Avocado Toast

Ingredients:

- 1 slice whole grain bread, toasted
- 1/2 ripe avocado
- Salt and pepper to taste
- Optional toppings: sliced tomatoes, sliced hard-boiled egg, or red pepper flakes

Instructions:

1. Mash the ripe avocado with a fork until smooth.
2. Spread mashed avocado evenly on the toasted whole-grain bread.
3. Season with salt and pepper.
4. Add optional toppings if desired.
5. Serve immediately.

Nutritional Information (per serving):

- Calories: 150
- Protein: 4g
- Fat: 10g

- Carbohydrates: 15g

Cottage Cheese with Pineapple

Ingredients:

- 1/2 cup cottage cheese
- 1/4 cup diced pineapple

Instructions:

1. Spoon cottage cheese into a bowl.
2. Top with diced pineapple.
3. Serve chilled.

Nutritional Information (per serving):

- Calories: 120
- Protein: 10g
- Fat: 2g
- Carbohydrates: 15g

Apple Slices with Almond Butter

Ingredients:

- 1 medium apple, sliced
- 2 tablespoons almond butter

Instructions:

1. Arrange apple slices on a plate.
2. Serve with almond butter for dipping.
3. Enjoy!

Nutritional Information (per serving):

- Calories: 200
- Protein: 4g
- Fat: 10g
- Carbohydrates: 25g

Hard-Boiled Eggs with Hummus

Ingredients:

- 2 hard-boiled eggs
- 2 tablespoons hummus
- Optional toppings: paprika, chopped parsley

Instructions:

1. Peel hard-boiled eggs and slice in half.
2. Serve with hummus for dipping.

3. Sprinkle with optional toppings if desired.

4. Serve chilled.

Nutritional Information (per serving):

- Calories: 160

- Protein: 12g

- Fat: 10g

- Carbohydrates: 6g

Trail Mix

Ingredients:

- 1/4 cup mixed nuts (almonds, cashews, walnuts)

- 1/4 cup dried fruit (raisins, cranberries, apricots)

- 2 tablespoons dark chocolate chips

Instructions:

1. Mix all ingredients in a bowl.

2. Portion into small snack bags for convenient grab-and-go snacks.

3. Enjoy!

Nutritional Information (per serving):

- Calories: 200
- Protein: 5g
- Fat: 12g
- Carbohydrates: 20g

Whole Grain Crackers with Cheese

Ingredients:

- 4 whole grain crackers
- 1 oz cheese (cheddar, Swiss, or your favorite variety)

Instructions:

1. Place crackers on a plate.
2. Top each cracker with a slice of cheese.
3. Serve immediately.

Nutritional Information (per serving):

- Calories: 200
- Protein: 8g

- Fat: 10g

- Carbohydrates: 15g

Vegetable Sticks with Hummus

Ingredients:

- 1/2 cup mixed vegetable sticks (carrots, celery, bell peppers)
- 2 tablespoons hummus

Instructions:

1. Arrange vegetable sticks on a plate.
2. Serve with hummus for dipping.
3. Enjoy!

Nutritional Information (per serving):

- Calories: 100
- Protein: 3g
- Fat: 5g
- Carbohydrates: 15g

Cucumber and Tomato Salad

Ingredients:

- 1/2 cucumber, sliced
- 1/2 cup cherry tomatoes, halved
- 1 tablespoon olive oil
- 1 tablespoon balsamic vinegar
- Salt and pepper to taste
- Fresh basil leaves for garnish

Instructions:

1. In a bowl, combine cucumber slices and halved cherry tomatoes.
2. Drizzle with olive oil and balsamic vinegar.
3. Season with salt and pepper.
4. Garnish with fresh basil leaves.
5. Serve chilled.

Nutritional Information (per serving):

- Calories: 80
- Protein: 1g
- Fat: 7g

- Carbohydrates: 5g

Greek Salad Skewers

Ingredients:

- Cherry tomatoes
- Cucumber, cut into chunks
- Black olives
- Feta cheese cut into cubes
- Wooden skewers

Instructions:

1. Thread cherry tomatoes, cucumber chunks, black olives, and feta cheese cubes onto wooden skewers.
2. Serve immediately.

Nutritional Information (per serving):

- Calories: 80
- Protein: 3g
- Fat: 5g
- Carbohydrates: 4g

Popcorn with Parmesan Cheese

Ingredients:

- 1/2 cup air-popped popcorn
- 1 tablespoon grated Parmesan cheese
- Optional: sprinkle of garlic powder or Italian seasoning

Instructions:

1. Pop popcorn according to package instructions.
2. Transfer popcorn to a bowl.
3. Sprinkle with grated Parmesan cheese.
4. Add optional seasonings if desired.
5. Toss gently to combine.
6. Enjoy!

Nutritional Information (per serving):

- Calories: 100
- Protein: 3g
- Fat: 3g

- Carbohydrates: 15g

Smoothie with Spinach and Berries

Ingredients:

- 1/2 cup fresh spinach leaves
- 1/2 cup mixed berries (strawberries, blueberries, raspberries)
- 1/2 cup Greek yogurt
- 1/2 cup unsweetened almond milk
- 1 tablespoon honey (optional)

Instructions:

1. Place spinach leaves, mixed berries, Greek yogurt, almond milk, and honey in a blender.
2. Blend until smooth.
3. Pour into a glass and serve immediately.

Nutritional Information (per serving):

- Calories: 150
- Protein: 10g

- Fat: 3g
- Carbohydrates: 20g

Chapter 10

ENDOMORPH DESSERT RECIPES

Baked Apples with Cinnamon

Ingredients:

- 2 apples, cored
- 1 tablespoon honey
- 1/2 teaspoon ground cinnamon

Instructions:

1. Preheat oven to 375°F (190°C).
2. Place cored apples in a baking dish.
3. Drizzle honey over the apples.
4. Sprinkle ground cinnamon over the apples.
5. Bake for 20-25 minutes or until apples are tender.
6. Serve warm.

Nutritional Information (per serving):

- Calories: 150
- Protein: 1g

- Fat: 0g
- Carbohydrates: 40g

Frozen Yogurt Bark

Ingredients:

- 1 cup Greek yogurt
- 1/4 cup mixed berries (strawberries, blueberries, raspberries)
- 2 tablespoons honey
- 2 tablespoons granola

Instructions:

1. Line a baking sheet with parchment paper.
2. Spread Greek yogurt evenly on the parchment paper.
3. Sprinkle mixed berries and granola over the yogurt.
4. Drizzle honey over the toppings.
5. Freeze for 2-3 hours or until firm.
6. Break into pieces and serve chilled.

Nutritional Information (per serving):

- Calories: 100

- Protein: 5g

- Fat: 2g

- Carbohydrates: 15g

Banana Oatmeal Cookies

Ingredients:

- 2 ripe bananas, mashed

- 1 cup rolled oats

- 1/4 cup chopped nuts (walnuts, almonds, or your choice)

- 1/4 cup dried fruit (raisins, cranberries, or your choice)

- 1 tablespoon honey

- 1 teaspoon ground cinnamon

Instructions:

1. Preheat oven to 350°F (175°C).
2. In a bowl, combine mashed bananas, rolled oats, chopped nuts,

dried fruit, honey, and ground cinnamon.

3. Drop spoonfuls of the mixture onto a baking sheet lined with parchment paper.

4. Flatten each spoonful with a fork.

5. Bake for 15-20 minutes or until golden brown.

6. Allow to cool before serving.

Nutritional Information (per serving):

- Calories: 120
- Protein: 3g
- Fat: 4g
- Carbohydrates: 20g

Chocolate Avocado Mousse

Ingredients:

- 1 ripe avocado
- 2 tablespoons cocoa powder
- 2 tablespoons honey

- 1/2 teaspoon vanilla extract
- Pinch of salt
- Optional toppings: sliced strawberries or raspberries

Instructions:

1. In a blender or food processor, combine ripe avocado, cocoa powder, honey, vanilla extract, and a pinch of salt.
2. Blend until smooth and creamy.
3. Transfer the mousse to serving bowls.
4. Chill in the refrigerator for at least 30 minutes.
5. Serve topped with sliced strawberries or raspberries if desired.

Nutritional Information (per serving):

- Calories: 200
- Protein: 3g
- Fat: 10g
- Carbohydrates: 25g

Baked Peaches with Greek Yogurt

Ingredients:

- 2 peaches, halved and pitted
- 1 tablespoon honey
- 1/4 teaspoon ground cinnamon
- 1/2 cup Greek yogurt

Instructions:

1. Preheat oven to 375°F (190°C).
2. Place peach halves, cut side up, in a baking dish.
3. Drizzle honey over the peaches.
4. Sprinkle ground cinnamon over the peaches.
5. Bake for 15-20 minutes or until peaches are tender.
6. Serve warm with a dollop of Greek yogurt.

Nutritional Information (per serving):

- Calories: 150
- Protein: 5g

- Fat: 0g

- Carbohydrates: 30g

Chia Seed Pudding

Ingredients:

- 1/4 cup chia seeds

- 1 cup unsweetened almond milk

- 1 tablespoon honey

- 1/2 teaspoon vanilla extract

- Optional toppings: sliced bananas, shredded coconut, or chopped nuts

Instructions:

1. In a bowl, mix chia seeds, almond milk, honey, and vanilla extract.

2. Cover and refrigerate for at least 2 hours or overnight, until the mixture thickens into a pudding-like consistency.

3. Stir well before serving.

4. Top with sliced bananas, shredded coconut, or chopped nuts if desired.

Nutritional Information (per serving):

- Calories: 150
- Protein: 5g
- Fat: 8g
- Carbohydrates: 15g

Fruit Salad with Honey-Lime Dressing

Ingredients:

- 1 cup mixed fruits (strawberries, kiwi, pineapple, grapes)
- 1 tablespoon honey
- Juice of 1 lime
- Fresh mint leaves for garnish

Instructions:

1. In a bowl, combine mixed fruits.
2. In a small bowl, whisk together honey and lime juice to make the dressing.

3. Drizzle the dressing over the fruit salad
    and toss gently to coat.

4. Garnish with fresh mint leaves.

5. Serve chilled.

Nutritional Information (per serving):

- Calories: 100

- Protein: 1g

- Fat: 0g

- Carbohydrates: 25g

Baked Pears with Almond Crumble

Ingredients:

- 2 pears, halved and cored

- 2 tablespoons almond flour

- 1 tablespoon rolled oats

- 1 tablespoon chopped almonds

- 1 tablespoon honey

- 1/4 teaspoon ground cinnamon

- Pinch of salt

Instructions:

1. Preheat oven to 375°F (190°C).
2. Place pear halves, cut side up, in a baking dish.
3. In a bowl, mix almond flour, rolled oats, chopped almonds, honey, ground cinnamon, and a pinch of salt to make the crumble topping.
4. Spoon the crumble mixture over the pear halves.
5. Bake for 20-25 minutes or until pears are tender and the crumble topping is golden brown.
6. Serve warm.

Nutritional Information (per serving):

- Calories: 200
- Protein: 3g
- Fat: 8g
- Carbohydrates: 30g

Coconut Chia Seed Popsicles

Ingredients:

- 1/4 cup chia seeds
- 1 cup coconut milk
- 2 tablespoons honey
- 1/2 teaspoon vanilla extract

Instructions:

1. In a bowl, mix chia seeds, coconut milk, honey, and vanilla extract.
2. Pour the mixture into popsicle molds.
3. Insert popsicle sticks into the molds.
4. Freeze for at least 4 hours or until firm.
5. Remove popsicles from molds and serve frozen.

Nutritional Information (per serving):

- Calories: 150
- Protein: 3g
- Fat: 10g
- Carbohydrates: 15g

Berry Parfait with Yogurt and Granola

Ingredients:

- 1/2 cup Greek yogurt
- 1/4 cup mixed berries (strawberries, blueberries, raspberries)
- 2 tablespoons granola

Instructions:

1. In a glass or bowl, layer Greek yogurt, mixed berries, and granola.
2. Repeat the layers.
3. Serve immediately.

Nutritional Information (per serving):

- Calories: 200
- Protein: 10g
- Fat: 3g
- Carbohydrates: 25g

Pumpkin Oatmeal Cookies

Ingredients:

- 1/2 cup canned pumpkin puree

- 1/2 cup rolled oats
- 1/4 cup almond flour
- 2 tablespoons honey
- 1/2 teaspoon ground cinnamon
- 1/4 teaspoon ground nutmeg
- 1/4 teaspoon ground ginger
- Pinch of salt

Instructions:

1. Preheat oven to 350°F (175°C).
2. In a bowl, mix pumpkin puree, rolled oats, almond flour, honey, ground cinnamon, ground nutmeg, ground ginger, and a pinch of salt.
3. Drop spoonfuls of the mixture onto a baking sheet lined with parchment paper.
4. Flatten each spoonful with a fork.
5. Bake for 15-20 minutes or until golden brown.

6. Allow to cool before serving.

Nutritional Information (per serving):

- Calories: 100
- Protein: 3g
- Fat: 3g
- Carbohydrates: 15g

Mango Coconut Rice Pudding

Ingredients:

- 1/2 cup cooked brown rice
- 1/2 cup coconut milk
- 1/4 cup diced mango
- 1 tablespoon honey
- 1/4 teaspoon vanilla extract

Instructions:

1. In a saucepan, combine cooked brown rice, coconut milk, diced mango, honey, and vanilla extract.

2. Cook over medium heat, stirring occasionally, until the mixture thickens into a pudding-like consistency.
3. Remove from heat and let cool slightly.
4. Serve warm or chilled.

Nutritional Information (per serving):

- Calories: 200
- Protein: 3g
- Fat: 10g
- Carbohydrates: 25g

Chapter 11

CONCLUSION

In conclusion, prioritizing a healthy weight and overall well-being holds paramount importance for seniors with endomorph body types. Embracing a well-rounded diet that prioritizes lean protein sources, beneficial fats, and complex carbohydrates while steering clear of processed foods and excessive sugars serves as a cornerstone for maintaining optimal weight and health. Moreover, integrating regular exercise into their lifestyle, encompassing both resistance training and cardiovascular activities, stands as a pivotal strategy to enhance muscle strength, fortify bone density, and foster cardiovascular wellness.

Given the unique physiological characteristics of endomorph seniors, it is imperative to acknowledge their specific needs and constraints. Consulting with a healthcare professional before embarking on any new dietary or exercise regimen is indispensable. Furthermore, ensuring adequate sleep and adopting effective stress management techniques are indispensable components of daily routines, bolstering overall health and well-being.

Through the consistent incorporation of wholesome habits into their daily lives, endomorph seniors can anticipate a range of benefits, including enhanced physical and cognitive functioning, mitigated risk of chronic ailments, and an elevated quality of life. This holistic approach not only nurtures their physical vitality but also nurtures their overall sense of fulfillment and contentment.